Babies
ANNE ENRIGHT

VINTAGE MINIS

Contents

Apologies All Round

SPEECH IS A selfish act, and mothers should probably remain silent. When one of these essays, about pregnancy, appeared in the *Guardian* magazine there was a ferocious response on the letters page. Who does she think she is? and Why should we be obliged to read about her insides? and Shouldn't she be writing about the sorrow of miscarriage instead?

So I'd like to say sorry to everyone in advance. Sorry. Sorry. Sorry. Sorry.

I'd like to apologise to all those people who find the whole idea of talking about things as opposed to just getting on with them mildly indecent, or provoking – I do know what they mean. Also to those who like to read about the dreadful things that happen to other people, when nothing particularly dreadful has happened to me, or my children, so far, touch wood, *Deo gratias*. Also to those readers who would prefer me not to think so much (because mothers just shouldn't), and to those thinkers who will realise that in the last few years I have not had time to research, or check a reference – the only books I have finished, since I had children, being the ones I wrote myself (not quite true, but it's a nice thing to say). And, of course, people who don't have children are just as good and fine and real as those who do, I would hate to imply otherwise. Also, sorry about my insides: I was reared with the idea that, for a woman, anatomy is destiny, so I have always paid close attention to what the body is and what it actually does. Call it a hobby.

'MARRIED WOMAN HAS CHILDREN IN THE SUBURBS' – it's not exactly a call to arms, and I do genuinely apologise for being so ordinary, in the worst sense. Here I am, all fortunate, living a 1950s ideal of baby powder and burps, except that, in the twenty-first century we know that talc is linked, bizarrely, to ovarian cancer, so there is no baby powder in this house, and we also know that the hand that rocks the cradle also pays for the cradle, or a fair amount of it, and that, for many people, babies are a luxury that they cannot yet afford. But even for the twenty-first century I am doing well: I have flexible working hours, no commuting, I have a partner who took six weeks off for the birth of his first baby and three months for the second (unpaid, unpaid, unpaid). He also does the breakfasts. And the baths. So you might well say, 'Oh, it's all right for her,' as I do when I read women writing about the problems they have with their nannies or other domestic staff. More usually, though, when I read women writing about having children, it is not their circumstances that annoy me so much as their tone. I think, 'What a wretch, would someone please call the social services.' It is the way they are both smug and astonished. It is the way we think we have done something amazing, when we have done no more than most other people on the planet – except we, in our over-educated way, have to brag about it.

Most of these pieces were started after my first child, a daughter, was born. I played around with them in the two years before I became pregnant again, and they were finished soon after the birth of my son, so though the baby is a 'she', both children are in there, somewhere. The reason I kept writing about my babies, even when they were asleep in the room, was that I could not think about anything else. This might account for any wildness of tone. The pieces were typed fast. They were written to the sound of a baby's sleeping breath. Some were assembled, later, from notes, but I have tried to keep the flavour of the original scraps.

Anyway, these are the material facts (for which I also apologise). I met my husband, Martin, a long time ago, we married I can't remember when, and after eighteen years of this and that we knuckled down to having children. It was not an impulse decision.

After our first child was born I worked while she slept, for the first year, and also in the evenings when her father came home. When she was one, she went to a nursery for (count them) six and a half hours per day, three of which were spent having a nap. When she was two and a half, she got a baby brother, and I worked while he slept. And so on. I would really like a rest, now.

Finally, and quietly, I have to apologise to my family and hope that they will forgive me for loving them in this formal, public, plundering way. Starting with my own mother – whose voice comes through my own, from time to time – and working down the generations. Like all women who write about their children, I have a wonderful partner – except in my case it is true. I also have to apologise to my children for writing about their baby selves; either too much, or not enough, or whatever changing way this book takes them, over the years.

My only excuse is that I think it is important. I wanted to say what it was like.

The Glass Wall

I SPENT MOST of my thirties facing a glass wall. On the other side of this wall were women with babies – 'mothers', you might call them. On my side were women who simply *were*. It didn't seem possible that I would ever move through the glass – I couldn't even imagine what it was like in there. All I could see were scattered reflections of myself; while on the other side real women moved with great slowness, like distantly sighted whales.

I always assumed I would have children, but only dimly – I never thought about when. I was reared in the seventies, by a woman who had been reared in the thirties, and we were both agreed that getting pregnant was the worst thing that could happen to a girl. My mother thought it would ruin my marriage prospects and I thought it would ruin my career prospects (same thing, really, by the different lights of our times). And when do you stop being a girl? By 'career' I meant something more than salary. I could not get pregnant, I thought, until I had 'gotten somewhere', until I 'knew who I was', until I was, in some way, more thoroughly myself.

These things are important: they do happen, but they often happen late, and you can hardly tell people to stop dithering. I look at women in their thirties with their noses pressed up against the glass, and all I can tell them (wave!) is that life in here on the other side is just the same – only much better, and more difficult.

I see them wondering, Does he love me and do I love him? and Will I have to give up smoking? and What about my job? and I don't want to be that fat woman in the supermarket, and What if it is autistic and Don't they cry all the time? and I want to say, 'It's fine.' More than that, when I first had a child, I was so delighted, I wanted to say, 'Do whatever it takes.' Children seemed to be such an absolute good, independent of the relationship that made them, that I wanted to say, 'Buy one if you have to,' or, 'Hurry.'

I was wrong, of course. Besides, most women are more interested in sexual love than they are in the maternal variety, they want a man more than they want children, or at least they want it *first*. Still, it is good to keep in mind the fact that, in a world where sexual partners can come and go, children remain. They are our enduring love.

It is good to keep in mind the fact that, in a world where sexual partners can come and go, children remain. They are our enduring love

Dream-Time

ONE FRIDAY IN October I started falling in love with everyone, and I stayed in love for two weeks, with everyone. This was awkward. It was a moony, teenage sort of love. I waited for the phone to ring. I was shy, almost anguished. I missed appointments, even with the people I loved, which was everyone, and so stayed at home and saw no one, my mind full of impossible thoughts.

I did manage to go to a school reunion (where I loved them all) and to the opening night of a play (where I made some wonderful new friends), but mostly I mooched, and wrote letters to celebrate the fact that I had just finished a book and that life was, perhaps unbearably, good.

Towards the end of this peculiar fortnight, I had a dream full of the usual suspects: people from my past who spoke to me in an unsettling, unresolved way. I have this dream, with variations, all the time, but this night it was interrupted by a woman I barely knew twenty years ago who floated in through a window, dressed in pink. She smiled an angelic smile, as if to say, 'None of this matters any more,' and then she patted her stomach, very gently. I started awake with the thought that I was pregnant; then I turned over to go back to sleep, saying to myself that the moment had come: it was time to stop the shilly-shally, the hit-and-miss, we had to get this conception thing going, properly, finally, and have the baby that was waiting for us, after all these years.

Soon after, I went to Berlin for a reading, half-dreading who I might be obliged to fall in love with there – but sometime in the middle of the weekend, I hit a wall. I couldn't say why this was. I didn't tell my hosts that I knew German and disliked the half-understood conversations they held in front of me, before turning to talk English with a smile. I walked the streets, planning a story about a woman who falls in love all the time, and another story that was full of mistranslation and sly insinuation, in which a woman meets a foreign couple and cannot quite tell what is going on.

My hostess said that she loved the passage in my book about a dream in which the ceiling is full of dangling penises. I have never written such a passage, nor anything like it, but she insisted: she was even quite insulted, as though I were accusing *her* of having my own pornographic thoughts. What could I say? I said I would check. But I noticed, in myself, a terrible physical weight, as if I could not carry my life around any more, I could not even lift it off the chair. I thought that perhaps I should stop writing books: something, at any rate, had to change. I walked from Schönhauser Allee to Unter den Linden, looking at the afternoon moon over Berlin, thinking that when it was full my period would come and then maybe everything would right itself again.

On the way back, I stopped over in London and got very drunk. The hangover seemed to last a week. I felt terrible. I dosed myself with miso soup and seaweed. I was insane for miso soup and seaweed. I still thought my life must change. I went on the Internet and typed in 'ovulation' on the search engine, then turned to my husband, Martin, saying, 'I think this beer is off. Is there something wrong with this beer?'

We bought the pregnancy test from a girl with romantic thoughts behind the cash register in Boots. Martin says I was delighted when it proved positive, but I was not delighted, I was shocked and delighted maybe, but I was mostly deeply shocked.

If Kafka had been a woman, then Gregor Samsa would not have turned into an insect, he would not have had to. Gregor would be Gretel and she would wake up one morning pregnant. She would try to roll over and discover she was stuck on her back. She would wave her little hands uselessly in the air.

It seems to me that I spent the next six weeks on the sofa listening to repeats of radio dramas, but my computer files record the fact that I worked, and that I also surfed the Net. I was looking for information on what happens when you get drunk in the very early stages of pregnancy, but the women on the Internet all wanted to lock expectant mothers up for drinking Diet Coke. In the chat rooms and on the notice-boards all the pregnant women talked about their pets: the cat who just knew, the dog who got upset. There was also a lot of stuff about miscarriages.

Martin took me up the mountains to keep me fit and I nearly puked into the bog. I got stuck on one tussock and could not jump to the next. The life inside me was too delicate, and impossible and small. No jumping, no running, no sex, no driving, no drink, no laughs, no household cleaning, no possibility, however vague or unwanted, of amorous adventures, no trips to India, no cheerful leaps from one tussock to the next in the god-damn bog. I made the jump anyway and went over on my ankle. Darkness started to fall.

The next weekend he brought me to Prague, as a surprise. There are two things in my life that I have never turned down, one is a drink and the other is an aeroplane ticket. Already, friends were starting to look askance when I stuck to water; now I sat in the departures lounge and did not want to board the plane. This intense reluctance, this exhaustion, was pregnancy. It was nine in the morning. People were running to the gates, buying newspapers, checking their boarding passes and drinking prophylactic shots of whiskey. I looked at the world around me and listened to my own blood. There was a deep note humming through me, so low that no one else could hear. It was in every part of me, swelling in my face and hands, and it felt like joy.

The weeks when you are generally, as opposed to locally, pregnant are a mess. I put on weight in odd places. I went to the kitchen in the middle of the night to see what nameless but really specific thing I was starving for. I sat down on the floor in front of the open fridge and cried. The aisles of the supermarket were filled with other possibly pregnant women – paralysed in front of the breakfast cereals, stroking packets of organic lentils, picking up, and setting down again, a six-pack of Petits Filous. Starvation is no joke, especially when you have been eating all day. I had, in my life, managed to have every neurosis except the one about food, and now my body was having it for me.

At ten weeks I went to the obstetrician, as if she could somehow fix what was wrong with me. We talked about postnatal depression (could I be having it already?). We talked about amniocentesis, but not much. She did not seem to realise that the child I had inside me would have to be deformed. She led me up a terrazzo staircase that smelt of school, and brought me into a dark room. 'Right,' she said, flicking on the light. 'Let's have a look.' I was expecting stirrups, but instead I got an ultrasound. The baby was like a little bean sprout. It flicked and jumped, as though annoyed to be disturbed. She lingered, with her sonic pen, as though this sight amazed her every time. It was all too much to bear. I said, 'It looks a bit disgusting,' and she said, 'Don't be silly,' as though she knew I was just shamming.

All of a sudden I was going to have a baby. The fact of my pregnancy was as real and constant to me as a con- crete block in the middle of the room, but I still did not know what it meant. A baby. A baby! I had to realise this many times: first with a premonition, then with a shock. I had to realise it slowly, and I had to realise the joy. After the ultrasound, it came to me all in a clatter and I walked home, roaring it out in my head. That night we went out to tell my parents. My mother said very little but, every time I looked at her, she looked five years younger, and then five years younger again. She was fundamentally, *metabolically* pleased. She was pleased all the way through, as I was pregnant all the way through.

I spent the next six months remembering and forget- ting again, catching up with what my body already knew. The world senses this gap. It seemed like everyone was trying to persuade me into this baby, as though they had made a great investment in me, and didn't trust me to take care of it. Out of badness, I did my best to drink (and failed) and took an occasional cigarette. This made one woman, a practical stranger, burst into tears. I wondered what her mother was like.

A pregnant woman is public property. I began to feel like a bus with 'Mammy' on the front – and the whole world was clambering on. Four women in a restaurant cheered when I ordered dessert. A friend went into a prolonged rage with me, for no reason at all. Everyone's unconscious was very close to their mouth. Whatever my pregnant body triggered was not social, or political, it was animal and ancient and quite helpless. It was also most unfair. Another friend showed me a pair of baby's shoes and said, 'Look, look!' He said that in prison, they show little shoes to child molesters to make them realise how small and vulnerable their victims were. He did not seem to notice that he had put pregnant women and child molesters in the same category, as if we both needed to be told what we were.

Perhaps he was right. A pregnant woman does not know what she is. She has been overtaken. She feels sick but she is not sick, she lives underwater, where there are no words. The world goes funny on her; it is accusing when she is delighted, and applauds when she feels like shit.

People without children went, without exception, a little mad. People who had children succumbed to a cherishing nostalgia. I began to enter into the romance of their lives, and see them as they must have been, newly married perhaps, and in love; dreaming of the future that they were living now. Pregnancy is a non-place, a suspension, a holiday from our fallible and compromised selves. There is no other time in a woman's life when she is so supported and praised and helped and loved. Though perhaps it is not 'she' who gets all the attention, but 'they'; this peculiar, mutant, double self – motherandchild.

I looked in the mirror. I had a body out of Rouault, big thick slabs of flesh, painted on stained glass. I was an amazement to myself, a work of engineering, my front cantilevered out from the solid buttress of my backside. Every night now, there was a ritual of wonder as we measured the bump. From week to week I felt my body shift into different cycles, like some slow-motion, flesh-based washing machine. 'Oh. Something else is happening now.' In the middle of January I surfaced, quite suddenly. I realised that the strenuous work was done, the baby was somehow 'made', all it had to do now was grow.

I have no idea why the first stages of pregnancy, when the child is so tiny, should be the most exhausting. I suppose you are growing your own cells before you start on theirs. Your blood volume goes up by 30 per cent, so your bone marrow is working, your very bone marrow is tired. It is as if you planted a seed and then had to build a field to grow it in. When that was over, everything, for me, was pure delight. If someone sold the hormones you get in the second trimester of pregnancy, I would become a junkie. I cycled everywhere, walked at a clip, fell asleep between one heartbeat and the next. I started dreaming again, vivid, intense, learning dreams. I was breast-feeding a blue-eyed girl and it was easy. I was in labour and it was easy – the child that slithered out was small and as hot as a childhood dream of wetting the bed; she was the precise temperature of flesh. Some of the dreams were funny, many were completely filthy. I had 30 per cent more blood

If someone sold the hormones you get in the second trimester of pregnancy, I would become a junkie

in my body and, as far as I could tell, it was all going to the one place. Another thing the books don't tell you.

The child was still hiding. The days ticked inexorably past. I did not feel like an animal, I felt like a clock, one made of blood and bone, that you could neither hurry nor delay. At four and a half months, right on cue, it started to chime. Butterflies. A kick.

The child leapt in my womb. Actually, the child leaps in the womb all day long, but it takes time for the womb to realise it. You wait for the first kick but, like the first smile, the early versions are all 'just wind'. The first definite kick (which coincided with the discovery of the first, definite pile, a shock severe enough to send a surge of adrenalin through any child) was wonderful. My body had been blind, and I barely comprehending; I had begun to long for a sign, a little something in return. The first kick is the child talking back to you, a kind of softening up. I began to have ideas about this baby, even conversations with it, some of which, to my great embarrassment, took place out loud.

'Hello, sweetheart.'

Sugar made the child jump, as well as hunger. Music made it stop, a listening stillness. I began to time my digestion: ten minutes after chocolate, a kick; fifteen minutes after pasta; half an hour after meat. I was bounced awake at five every morning and got up for a bowl of cereal – already feeding this little tyrant, getting in training for the real event. Early afternoon was a cancan, also nine o'clock at night. I went to New York and the child stayed on Irish time, which was very odd. In the middle of the day I would go back to my hotel room for a rest and a chat. My belly made peculiar company. We watched *My Dinner with Andre* together, and ate big handfuls of nuts.

What did I know? I knew this child liked music, but maybe all children do. I thought it was an independent type, wriggling already, as though to get away. I began to identify whatever part of its body was squirming under my hand. One day a shoulder bone scything up from the depths, another day a little jutting heel. My indifference to the world grew vast. I liked things from a distance. I was in the middle of the sweetest, quietest romance.

In our first antenatal class the midwife said, 'Is there a pelvis over there on the floor behind you, could you pass it here?' And when some hapless male picked up the bit of dead person they used for demonstration purposes, she said, 'Don't be afraid of it. It's not a chalice.' I thought this was very Irish. Secretly, I thought that perhaps my pelvis *was* a chalice. I also thought that it might be beginning to crack. She passed around a vial of amniotic fluid (of unspecified age, it would have been nice to know if it was fresh) and on the other side of the room, a woman bent forward on to her belly, in an awkward, pregnant attempt at a faint. The midwife turned to a diagram – we had to have the window opened for air. She told us about perineal mas-sage. I had never heard of anything so peculiar and unlikely in my life. I was surrounded by strangers, half of them men and all of them catatonic with shock. It might have been the way she lay down on a mat with her legs up in the air (she was in her late fifties), or it might just have been the fact that all of us realised that there was a fundamental problem, here, of design. The hole just wasn't big enough. And there was no escape now. I felt as though I had been watching a distant train for months and only now, when it was approaching, did I realise I was tied to the tracks.

My father says, quite wisely, that we should have been marsupials, pregnant up to six months, with the last three in a pouch. The disproportion was terrible. This could not be what nature intended, humans must be overbred. I couldn't walk for more than twenty minutes. Everything hurt. Somehow, I blamed the bump and not the child for the obstruction in my gut and the vile acid that was pushed up into my throat. We weren't to take antacids, because they would make us anaemic, the midwife said. I said, 'What's so bad about anaemia?' thinking that it couldn't be worse than this. I sat and surfed the Net like some terrible turnip, gagging and leaning back in my chair. My shoes didn't fit. I became clumsy, and not just because of the weight out front – dishes dropped for no reason out of my hands. At thirty-five weeks, just like all the other women on the About.com pregnancy notice-board, I started fighting with Martin: even this was predetermined, as the hormonal conveyor belt ground on. Oh, the stupidity of it, the blankness, the senseless days and the terrible, interrupted nights. Somewhere in there, I forgot entirely that I was having a child. Nothing wonderful could come of this.

I was bored to madness, and there was nothing I, or anyone else, could do about it because I had the concentration span of a gnat. A very fat gnat.

The streets, that had been full of babies in their buggies, now became full of the old and the infirm, people who couldn't manage the step on to the bus, or who failed to reach the queue before the till closed. Was it possible that pregnancy was turning me into a nicer person? I thought of the women I knew when I was young who were pregnant all the time. I did sums: the mother of a school friend who had had twenty-two pregnancies, eleven of which had come to term. She would look up from her plate, surrounded by bottles of pills, and say, 'Oh . . . Hello . . .' as though trying to figure out if you had come out of her or someone else. Her husband was mad about her, you could still see it, and her children, with the exception of the eldest boys, were complete strangers.

Even my own much discussed, often caressed, high-focus bump was filled with someone I did not know. And perhaps never would. Pregnancy is as old-fashioned as religion, and it never ends. Every moment of my pregnancy lasted for ever. I was pregnant in the autumn, and I was pregnant in the spring. I was pregnant as summer came. I lived like a plant on the window-sill, taking its time, starting to bud. Nothing could hurry this. There was no technology for it: I was the technology – increasingly stupid, increasingly kind, a mystery to myself, to Martin, and to everyone who passed me by.

Birth

AMNIOTIC FLUID SMELLS like tea. When I say this to Martin, he says, 'I thought that was just tea.' Of course a hospital should smell of tea: a hospital should smell of bleach. Unit C smells of tea and a little bit of ammonia, whether human or industrial is hard to tell. There is a lot of amniotic fluid in Unit C. At least three of the women have had their waters broken that afternoon, and as the evening approaches we sit draining into strips of unbleached cotton and watching each other, jealously, for signs of pain.

There is a little something extra in there, sharp and herbal – green tea maybe, or gunpowder tea. Pregnancy smelt like grass. Sort of. It certainly smelt of something growing; a distinctive and lovely smell that belongs to that family of grass, and ironed cotton, and asparagus pee. But the smell of tea is beginning to get to me. There are pints of it. I'm like some Burco Boiler with the tap left open. It flows slowly, but it will not stop. For hours I have been waiting for it to stop, and the mess of the bed is upsetting me. It upsets the housekeeper in me and it upsets the schoolgirl in me. The sanitary pads they hand you are school-issue and all the nurses are turning into nuns.

The breaking of the waters was fine. The nurse did whatever magic makes sheets appear under you while other things are folded back, and the obstetrician did something deft with a crochet hook. There was the sense of pressure against a membrane, and then pop – a bit tougher but not much different from bursting a bubble on plastic bubble wrap. It felt quite satisfying, and the rush of hot liquid that followed made me laugh. I don't think a lot of women laugh at this stage in Unit C, but why not? We were on our way.

After which, there is nothing to do but wait. As the afternoon wears on, the pink curtains are pulled around the beds. The ward is full of breathing; the sharp intake of breath and the groaning exhalation, as though we are all asleep, or having sex in our sleep. One woman sobs behind her curtain. From the bed beside me the submarine sound of the Doppler looking for a foetal heartbeat and endlessly failing – a sonic rip as it is pulled away, then bleeping, breathing; the sigh and rush of an unseen woman's electronic blood.

Then there is tea. Actual tea. The men are sent out, for some reason, and the women sit around the long table in the middle of the ward. It's a school tea. There is a woman with high blood pressure, a couple of diabetics, one barely pregnant woman who has such bad nausea she has to be put on a drip. There are at least three other women on the brink, but they stay in bed and will not eat. I am all excited and want to talk. I am very keen to compare dressing-gowns – it took me so long to find this one, and I am quite pleased with it, but when I get up after the meal, the back of it is stained a watery red. I am beginning to hate Unit C.

After tea is the football. Portugal are playing France and, when a goal is scored, the men all come out from behind the curtains to watch the replay. Then they go back in again to their groaning, sighing women. I keep the curtain open and watch Martin while he watches the game. I am keeping track of my contractions, if they are contractions. At 9.35, Martin looks at me over the back of his chair. He gives me a thumbs-up as if to say, 'Isn't this a blast? And there's football on the telly!' At 9.35 and 20 seconds I am, for the first time, in serious pain. I am in a rage with him for missing it, and call to him quietly over the sound of the game.

A woman in a dressing-gown comes to talk to me. She is very big. I ask her if she is due tonight but she says she is not due until September, which is three months away. She is the woman from the next bed, the one with the Doppler machine. They couldn't find the foetal heartbeat because of the fat. She stands at the end of the bed and lists her symptoms, which are many. She has come up from Tipperary. She is going to have a Caesarean at thirty-one weeks. I am trying to be sympathetic, but I think I hate her. She is weakness in the room.

When I have a contraction I lurch out of bed, endlessly convinced that I have to go to the toilet – endlessly, stupidly convinced, every five minutes, that there is a crap I have to take, new and surprising as the first crap Adam took on his second day in the world. This journey to the toilet is full of obstacles, the first one being Martin, whose patience is endless and whose feet are huge. When I get into the cubicle at the end of the ward, I sit uselessly on the toilet, try to mop up the mess, and listen to the woman on the other side of the partition, who is louder than me, and who doesn't seem to bother going back to her bed any more.

This has been happening, on and off, for a week. There is nothing inside me by way of food; there hasn't been for days. I am in what Americans call pre-labour, what the Irish are too macho to call anything at all. 'If you can talk through it, then it's not a contraction,' my obstetrician said when I came in a week ago, convinced that I was on my way. This week, she says, she will induce me because my blood pressure is up; but it may be simple charity. Ten days ago I wanted a natural birth, now I want a general anaesthetic. Fuck aromatherapy, I would do anything to make this stop – up to, and including, putting my head in the road, with my belly up on the kerb.

A woman answers her mobile, 'No, Ma, nothing yet. Stop calling! Nothing yet.' Pain overtakes the woman two beds down and the curtains are drawn. When they are pulled back, you can tell she is delighted. Oh, this is it. This *must* be it. Oh, oh, I'm going to have a baby. Then more pain – agony, it looks like. 'Oh, good girl! Good girl!' shouts the midwife, as the man collects her things and she is helped out of the Ante-Room to Hell that is Unit C. I am jealous, but I wish her well. The room is full of miracles waiting to happen, whether months or hours away. Another bed is empty – the woman on the other side of the toilet partition, is she in labour too? 'She went out, anyway,' says Martin. 'Hanging on to the wall.'

It is a theatre of pain. It is a pain competition (and I am losing). Martin says that Beckett would have loved Unit C. We wonder whether this is the worst place we have ever been, but decide that the prize still goes to the bus station in Nasca, the time we went to Peru and didn't bring any jumpers. All the paper pants I brought have torn and I sit knickerless on the unbleached sheet, which I have rolled up into a huge wad under me. My bump has shrunk a little, and gone slack. When I put my hand on it, there is the baby; very close now under the skin. I just know it is a girl. I feel her shoulder and an arm. For some reason I think of a skinned rabbit. I wonder are her eyes open, and if she is waiting, like me. I have loved this child in a drowsy sort of way, but now I feel a big want in me for her, for this particular baby – the one that I am touching through my skin. 'Oh, when will I see you?' I say.

This could be the phrase of the night, but instead it is

a song that repeats in my head. 'What sends her home hanging on to the wall? Boozin'! Bloody well boo-oozin'.' I stop getting out of bed every five minutes and start breathing, the way they told us to in the antenatal class. I count backwards from five when the pain hits, and then from five again. Was I in labour yet? Was this enough pain? 'If you can talk, then it's not labour.' So I try to keep talking, but by 11.00 the lights are switched off, I am lurching into sleep between my (non-)contractions for three or five minutes at a time, and Martin is nodding off in the chair.

My cervix has to do five things: it has to come forward, it has to shorten, it has to soften, it has to thin out, it has to open. A week earlier the obstetrician recited this list and told me that it had already done three of them. In the reaches of the night I try to remember which ones I have left to do, but I can't recall the order they come in, and there is always, as I press my counting fingers into the sheet, one that I have forgotten. My cervix, my cervix. Is it soft but not short? Is it soft and thin, but not yet forward? Is it short and hard, but open anyway? I have no sense that this is not a list but a sequence. I have lost my grasp of cause and effect. My cervix, my cervix: it will open as the clouds open, to let the sun come shining through. It will open like the iris of an eye, like the iris when you open the back of a camera. I could see it thinning; the tiny veins stretching and breaking. I could see it opening like something out of *Alien*. I could see it open as simply as a door that you don't know you've opened, until you are halfway across the room. I could see all this, but my cervix stayed shut.

At 2.30 a.m. I give in and Martin goes off to ask for some Pethidine. I know I will only be allowed two doses of this stuff, so it had better last a long time. I want to save the second for the birth, but in my heart of hearts I know I'm on my way to an epidural now. I don't know why I wanted to do without one, I suppose it was that Irish-woman machismo again. *Mná na hEireann. MNÁ na hEireann.* FIVE four three two . . . one. Fiiiive four three two one. Five. Four. Three. Two. One.

Once I give in and start to whimper, the (non-)contractions are unbearable. The Pethidine does not come. At 3 a.m. there is a shrieking from down the corridor, and I realise how close we are to the labour ward. The noise is ghastly, Victorian: it tears through the hospital dark. Someone is really giving it soprano. I think nothing of it. I do not wonder if the woman is mad, or if the baby has died, but that is what I wonder as I write this now.

Footsteps approach but they are not for me, they are for the woman from Tipperary who has started crying, with a great expenditure of snot, in the bed next door. The nurse comforts her. 'I'm just frikened,' the woman says. 'She just frikened me.' I want to shout that it's all right for her, she's going to have a fucking Caesarean, but it has been forty-five minutes since I realised that I could not do this any more, that the pain I had been riding was about to ride over me, and I needed something to get me back on top, or I would be destroyed by it, I would go under – in some spiritual and very real sense, I would die.

The footsteps go away again. They do not return. I look at Martin who is listening, as I am listening, and he disappears silently through the curtain. At 3.30 a.m., I get the Pethidine.

After this, I do not count through the (non-)contractions, or try to manage my breathing. I moan, with my mouth a little open. I *low*. I almost enjoy it. I sleep all the time now, between times. I have given in. I have untied my little boat and gone floating downstream.

At 5.00 a.m. a new woman comes along and tells Martin he must go home. There follows a complicated and slow conversation as I stand up to her (we are, after all, back in school). I say that I need him here, and she smiles, 'What for? What do you need him for?' (For saving me from women like you, *Missus*.) In the end, she tells us that there are mattresses he can sleep on in a room down the hall. Oh. Why didn't she say so? Maybe she's mad. It's 5 a.m., I'm tripping on Pethidine, at the raw end of a sleepless week, and this woman is a little old-fashioned, in a mad sort of way. Wow. We kiss. He goes. From now on, I stay under, not even opening my eyes when the pain comes.

I think I low through breakfast. They promise me a bed in the labour ward at 10.30, so I can stop lowing and start screaming, but that doesn't seem to be happening really.

I am sitting up and smiling for the ward round, which is nice, but I am afraid that they will notice that the contractions are fading, and I'll have to start all over again, somehow. Then the contractions come back again, and by now my body is all out of Pethidine. I spend the minutes after 10.30 amused by my rage; astonished by how bad I feel. Are these the worst hundred seconds I have ever been through? How about the next hundred seconds – let's give them a go.

At 12.00, I nip into the cubicle for one last contraction, and we are out of Unit C. The whole ward lifts as we leave, wishing us well – another one on her way. I realise I have been lowing all night, keeping these women from sleep.

The room on the labour ward is extremely posh, with its own bathroom and a high-tech bed. I like the look of the midwife; she is the kind of woman you'd want to go for a few pints with. She is tired. She asks if I have a birth plan and I say I want to do everything as naturally as possible. She says, 'Well, you've made a good start, anyway,' which I think is possibly sarcastic, given the crochet hook, and the Pethidine, and the oxytocin drip they've just ordered up. Martin goes back to pack up our stuff, and I start to talk. She keeps a half-ironic silence. For months, I had the idea that if I could do a bit of research, get a bit of chat out of the midwife, then that would take my mind off things – what is the worst thing that anyone ever said? or the weirdest? – but she won't play ball. I run out of natter and have a little cry. She says, 'Are you all right?' I say, 'I just didn't think I would ever get this far, that's all.' And I feel her soften behind me.

I don't remember everything that followed, but I do remember the white, fresh light. I also remember the feelings in the room. I could sense a shift in mood, or intention, in the women who tended me, with great clarity. It was like being in a painting. Every smile mattered; the way people were arranged in the space, the gestures they made.

I have stopped talking. The midwife is behind me, arranging things on a stand. Martin is gone, there is silence in the room. She is thinking about something. She isn't happy. It is very peaceful.

Or: She tries to put in the needle for the drip. Martin is on my right-hand side. I seem to cooperate but I won't turn my hand around. The stain from the missed vein starts to spread and she tries again. I am completely uninterested in the pain from the needle.

Or: A woman walks in, looks at me, glances between my legs. 'Well done!' she says, and walks back out again. Perhaps she just walked into the wrong room.

Even at a low dose, the oxytocin works fast. It is bucking through my system, the contractions gathering speed: the donkey who is kicking me is getting really, really annoyed. The midwife goes to turn up the drip and I say, 'You're not touching that until I get my epidural.' A joke.

A woman puts her head round the door, then edges into the room. She says something to the midwife, but they are really talking about something else. She half-turns to me with a smile. There is something wrong with one of the blood tests. She tells me this, then she tells the midwife that we can go ahead anyway. The midwife relaxes. I realise that, sometimes, they don't give you an epidural. Even if you want one. They just can't. Then everyone has a bad morning.

The midwife goes to the phone. Martin helps to turn me on my side. The contractions now are almost continuous. Within minutes, a woman in surgical greens walks in. 'Hi!' she says. 'I'm your pain-relief consultant.' She reaches over my bare backside to shake my hand. This is a woman who loves her job. Martin cups my heels and pushes my knees up towards my chest, while she sticks the needle in my spine, speaking clearly and loudly, and working at speed. I am bellowing by now, pretty much. FIVE, I roar (which seems to surprise them – five what?) FOUR. THREE. (Oh, good woman! That's it!) TWO. One. FIVE. They hold me like an animal that is trying to kick free, but I am not – I am doing this, I am getting this done. When it is over, the anaesthetist breaks it to me that it might be another ten minutes before I feel the full effect. I do not have ten minutes to spare, I want to tell her this, but fortunately, the pain has already begun to dull.

The room turns to me. The anaesthetist pats down her gown and smiles. She is used to the most abject gratitude, but I thank the midwife instead, for getting the timing spot on. The woman who talked about my blood tests has come back and the midwife tells me that she is finishing up now, Sally will see me through. This is a minor sort of betrayal, but I feel it quite keenly. Everyone leaves. Martin goes for a sandwich and Sally runs ice-cubes up my belly to check the line of the epidural. There is no more pain.

Sally is lovely: sweetness itself. She is the kind of woman who is good all the way through. It is perhaps 1.30 and in the white light, with no pain, I am having the time of my life. Literally. Karen, the obstetrician, tells me my cervix has gone from practically 0 to 8 centimetres, in no time flat. The heavens have opened, the sun has come shining through. Martin is called back from the canteen. He watches the machines as they register the pain that I cannot feel any more. He says the contractions are off the scale now. We chat a bit and have a laugh, and quite soon Sally says it is time to push. Already.

For twenty hours women have been telling me I am wonderful, but I did not believe them until now. I know how to do this, I have done it in my dreams. I ask to sit up a bit and the bed rises with a whirr. Martin is invited to 'take a leg' and he politely accepts, 'Oh, thank you.' Sally takes the other one, and braces it – my shin against her ribs. Push! They both lean into me. I wait for the top of the contraction, catch it, and ride the wave. I can feel the head, deliciously large under my pubic bone. I can feel it as it eases further down. I look at Martin, all the while – here is a present for you, mister, this one is for you – but he is busy watching the business end. Karen is back, and they are all willing me on like football hooligans, Go on! Go on! One more now, and Push! Good woman! Good girl! I can hear the knocking of the baby's heartbeat on the foetal monitor, and the dreadful silence as I push. Then, long before I expect it, Sally says, 'I want you to pant through this one. Pant.' The child has come down, the child is there. Karen says, Yes, you can see the head. I send Martin down to check the colour of the hair. (A joke?) Another push. I ask may I touch, and there is the top of the head, slimy and hot and – what is most terrifying – soft. Bizarrely, I pick up Martin's finger to check that it is clean, then tell him he must feel how soft it is. So he does. After which – enough nonsense now – it is back to pushing. Sally reaches in with her flat-bladed scissors and Martin, watching, lets my leg go suddenly slack. We are mid-push. I kick out, and he braces against me again. Karen, delighted, commands me to, 'Look down now, and see your baby being born.' I tilt my head to the maximum; and there is the back of the baby's head, easing out beyond my belly's horizon line. It is black and red, and wet. On the next push, machine perfect, it slowly turns. And here it comes – my child; my child's particular profile. A look of intense concentration, the nose tilted up, mouth and eyes tentatively shut. A blind man's face, vivid with sensation. On the next push, Sally catches the shoulders and lifts the baby out and up – in the middle of which movement the mouth opens, quite simply, for a first breath. It simply starts to breathe.

'It's a girl!'

Sally says afterwards that we were very quiet when she came out. But I didn't want to say the first thing that came to mind – which was, 'Is it? Are you sure?' A newborn's genitals are swollen and red and a bit peculiar looking, and the cord was surprisingly grey and twisted like a baroque pillar. Besides, I was shy. How to make the introduction? I think I eventually said, 'Oh, I knew you would be,' I think I also said, 'Oh, come here to me, darling.' She was handed to me, smeared as she was with something a bit stickier than cream cheese. I laid her on my stomach and pulled at my T-shirt to clear a place for her on my breast. She opened her eyes for the first time, looking into my face, her irises cloudy. She blinked and found my eyes. It was a very suspicious, grumpy look, and I was devastated.

Martin, doing the honours at a festive dinner, cut the cord. After I pushed out the placenta, Karen held it up for inspection, twirling it on her hand like a connoisseur: a bloody hairnet, though heavier and more slippy.

The baby was long. Her face looked like mine. I had not prepared myself for this: this really astonished me. 'She looks like me.' And Martin said (an old joke), 'But she's got my legs.' At some stage, she was wrapped rigid in a blue blanket, which was a mercy, because I could hardly bear the smallness of her. At some stage, they slipped out, leaving us to say, 'Oh, my God,' a lot. I put her to a nipple and she suckled. 'Oh, my *God*,' said Martin. I looked at him as if to say, 'Well, what did you expect?' I rang my mother who said, 'Welcome to the happiest day of your life,' and started to cry. I thought this was a little over the top. In a photograph taken at this time, I look pragmatic and unsurprised, as though I had just cleaned the oven and was about to tackle the fridge.

I am not stricken until they wheel us down to the ward. The child looks at the passing scene with alert pleasure. She is so clear and sharp. She is saturated with life, she is intensely alive. Her face is a little triangle and her eyes are shaped like leaves, and she looks out of them, liking the world.

Two hours later I am in the shower. When I clean between my legs I am surprised to find everything numb and mushy. I wonder why that is. Then I remember that a baby's head came out of there, actually came out. When I come to, I am sitting on a nurse. She is sitting on the toilet beside the shower. The shower is still going. I am very wet. She is saying, 'You're all right, you're all right, I've got you.' I think I am saying, 'I just had a baby. I just had a baby,' but I might be trying to say it, and not saying anything at all.

Milk

THE MILK SURPRISES me. It does not disgust me as much as I thought it would, unless it is not fresh. It is disturbing that a piece of you should go off so quickly. I don't think Freud ever discussed lactation, but the distinction between 'good' and 'bad' bodily products here is very fine. Women leak so much. Perhaps this is why we clean – which is to say that a man who cleans is always 'anal', a woman who cleans is just a woman.

There certainly is a lot of it, and it gets everywhere, and the laundry is a fright. But what fun! to be granted a new bodily function so late in life. As if you woke up one morning and could play the piano. From day to day the child is heavier in your arms, she plumps up from wrist to ankle, she has dimples where her knuckles were, she has fat on her toes. I thought we might trade weight, pound for pound, but she is gaining more than I am losing. I am faced with bizarre and difficult calculations – the weight of the groceries in a bag versus the weight of her nappies in a bag. Or my weight, plus a pint of water, minus four ounces of milk, versus her weight, plus four ounces, divided by yesterday. When I was at school, a big-chested friend put her breasts on the scales and figured that they weighed 2 pounds each. I don't know how she did it, but I still think that she was wrong. Heavier. Much heavier.

It is quite pleasant when a part of your body makes sense, after many years. A man can fancy your backside, but you still get to sit on it; breasts, on the other hand, were always just there. Even so, the anxiety of pregnancy is the anxiety of puberty all over again. I am thirty-seven. I don't want my body to start 'doing' things, like some kind of axolotl. I do not believe people when they say these things will be wonderful, that they are 'meant'. I am suspicious of the gleam in women's eyes, that pack of believers, and listen instead to the voice of a friend who breast-fed her children until they were twenty-eight years old, and who now says, 'They're like ticks.'

So I feed the child because I should, and resign myself to staying home. I never liked being around nursing women – there was always too much love, too much need in the room. I also suspected it to be sexually gratifying. For whom? Oh, for everyone: for the mother, the child, the father, the father-in-law. Everyone's voice that little bit nervy, as though it weren't happening: everyone taking pleasure in a perv-lite middle-class sort of way. Ick. 'The only women who breast-feed are doctors' wives and tinkers,' a friend's mother was told forty years ago, by the nurse who delivered her. I thought I sensed a similar distaste in the midwives, a couple of months ago, who were obliged by hospital and government policy to prod the child and pinch my nipple, though perhaps – let's face it, sisters – not quite that hard. It is probably easier for men, who like breasts in general, but I have always found them mildly disgusting, at least up close. They also often make me jealous. Even the word 'breast' is difficult. Funny how many people say they find public breast-feeding a bit 'in your face'. Oh, the rage.

So, let us call it 'nursing' and let us be discreet – it is still the best way I know to clear a room. My breast is not the problem (left, or right, whichever is at issue), the 'problem' is the noise. Sometimes the child drinks as simply as from a cup, other times she snorts and gulps, half-drowns, sputters and gasps; then she squawks a bit, and starts all over again. This may be an iconised activity made sacred by some and disgusting by others, but it is first and foremost a meal. It is only occasionally serene. It also takes a long time. I do smile at her and coo a bit, but I also read a lot (she will hate books), talk, or type (this, for example). Afterwards she throws up. People stare at the whiteness of it, as I did at first. Look. Milk.

'It was the whiteness of the whale that above all appalled me.' The nineteenth century took their breasts very seriously, or so I suspect – I can't really get into a library to check. I am thinking of those references I found particularly exciting or unsettling as a child. The heroes of *King Solomon's Mines*, for example, as they toil up She-ba's left Breast (a mountain) suffering from a torturing thirst. The chapter is called 'Water Water!' and comes from a time when you were allowed to be so obvious it hurt. 'Heavens, how we did drink!' These extinct volca-noes are 'inexpressibly solemn and overpowering' and difficult to describe. They are wreathed about with 'strange mists and clouds [that] gathered and increased around them, till presently we could only trace their pure and gigantic outline swelling ghostlike through the fleecy envelope'. In a desperate drama of hunger and satiation our heroes climb through lava and snow up to the hill-ock of the enormous, freezing nipple. There they find a cave, occupied by a dead man (what?! what?!), and in this cave one of their party also dies: Ventvogel, a 'hottentot' whose 'snub-nose' had, when he was alive, the ability to sniff out water (we don't want to know).

So far, so infantile. I watch the child's drama at the breast, and (when I am not reading, typing, or talking) cheer her along. She wakes with a shout in the middle of the night, and I wonder at her dreams; there is a dead man in a cave, perhaps, somewhere about my person. Oh, dear. When did it all get so serious? I turn to Swift for the com-edy, as opposed to tragedy, of scale, but Gulliver perched on a Brobdingnagian nipple turns out, on rereading, to be part of a great disgustfest about giant women pissing. None of this seems *true* to me. I have no use for the child's disgust, as she has no use for mine. I am besotted by a being who is, at this stage, just a set of emotions arranged around a gut. Who is just a shitter, who is just a soul.

Are all mothers Manicheans? This is just one of the hundreds of questions that have never been asked about motherhood. What I am interested in is not the drama of being a child, but this new drama of being a mother (yes, there are cannibals in my dreams, yes) about which so little has been written. Can mothers not hold a pen? Or is it just the fact that we are all children, when we write?

I go to Books Upstairs in Dublin, to find a poem by Eavan Boland. The child in the stroller is ghetto fabulous in a white babygro complete with hoodie. I am inordinately, sadly proud of the fact that she is clean. We negotiate the steps, we knock over some books. The child does a spectacular crap in the silence of the shop, in front of the section marked 'Philosophy'. I say, 'Oh, look at all the books. Oh, *look* at all the books,' because I believe in talking to her, and I don't know what else to say.

The poem is called 'Night Feed' and is beautifully measured and very satisfying: 'A silt of milk. / The last suck. / And now your eyes are open, / Birth coloured and offended.'

But the poet chooses a bottle not a breast, placing the poem in the bland modernity of the suburbs. I grew up in those suburbs. I know what we were running away from. Because the unpalatable fact is that the Ireland of my childhood had the closest thing to a cow cult outside of India. When I was eleven, I won a Kodak Instamatic camera in the Milk Competition, a major annual event, when every school child in the country had to write an essay called 'The Story of Milk'. I can still remember the arrival of the Charolais cattle, which marked the beginning of Ireland's love affair with Europe. The most exciting thing about economic union, for my farming relatives, was not the promise of government grants but this big-eyed, nougat-coloured breed of bull whose semen could be used in beef or dairy herds – as good, if you will pardon the phrase, for meat as for milk. It was a romantic animal, as hopeful as the moon shot. There were cuff-links made in the shape of the Charolais and men wore them to Mass and to the mart. And the romance lingers on. A couple of years ago, a media personality of my acquaintance bought four of them, to match her curtains.

The country was awash with milk. Kitchens and bedrooms were hung with pictures of the Madonna and child. After the arrival of infant formula in the fifties, breast-feeding became more of a chosen, middle-class activity, but it was still common in the countryside, and was everywhere practised as a fairly optimistic form of contraception. Still, though general all over Ireland, breast-feeding was absolutely hidden. The closest the culture came to an image of actual nursing was in the icon of the Sacred Heart, endlessly offering his male breast, open and glowing, and crowned with thorns.

Actually, you know, breast-feeding hurts. Certainly, at first, it really fucking hurts. On the third night of my daughter's life I was left with a human being the size of a cat and nothing to sustain her with but this *stub*. Madwomen (apparently) think that their babies are possessed. And they are. They look at you, possessed by their own astonishing selves. You say, Where did that come from? You say, Where did YOU come from? This baby is pure need – a need you never knew you had. And all you have to offer is a mute part of your body which, you are told, will somehow start 'expressing', as though it might start singing 'Summertime'. You feed your child, it seems, on hope alone. There is nothing to see. You do not believe the milk exists until she throws it back up, and when she does, you want to cry. What is not quite yours as it leaves you, is definitely yours as it comes back.

So there we were in the hospital dark; me and my white Dracula, her chin running with milk and her eyes black. What I remember is how fully human her gaze was, even though it was so new. She seemed to say that this was a serious business, that we were in it together. Tiny babies have such emotional complexity. I am amazed that 'bravery' is one of the feelings she has already experienced, that she should be born so intrepid and easily affronted, that she should be born so much herself.

She is also, at this early stage, almost gender free. This is useful. The statistics on how much less girl babies are breast-fed, as opposed to boys, are shocking. There are probably a number of reasons for this, but one of them surely is the degree to which our society has sexualised the breast. All in all, sex has ruined breast-feeding. It is a moral business these days – a slightly dirty, slightly wonderful, always unsettling, duty. It has no comic aspects. No one has told the child this: she seems to find it, finally, quite amusing – as indeed do I.

We turn to Sterne to find glee, envy, all those ravening eighteenth-century emotions, transmuted by language into delight. Shandy quotes Ambrose Paraeus on the stunting effect of the nursing breast on a child's nose, particularly those 'organs of nutrition' that have 'firmness and elastic repulsion'. These were 'the undoing of the child, inasmuch as his nose was so snubb'd, so rebuff'd, so rebated, and so refrigerated thereby, as never to arrive ad mensuram suam legitimam'. What was needed was a soft, flaccid breast so that, 'by sinking into it . . . as into so much butter, the nose was comforted, nourish'd, plump'd up, refresh'd, refocillated, and set a growing for ever'.

This was still when 'breast' was a common, easy word. Men placed their hands on their breasts, had pistols pointed at them, and were in general so set to a-swelling and a-glowing as to put the girls to shame. There is a distinction between 'breast' and 'breasts', of course, but it is still charming to think that this seat of honesty and sentiment is the singular of a plural that provoked desire. As if, in modern terms, we got horny watching someone's eyes fill with tears. As, indeed, sometimes, we do.

No. The milk surprises me, above all, because it hurts as it is let down, and this foolish pain hits me at quite the wrong times. The reflex is designed to work at the sight, sound, or thought of your baby – which is spooky enough – but the brain doesn't seem to know what a baby *is*, exactly, and so tries to make you feed anything helpless, or wonderful, or small. So I have let down milk for Russian submariners and German tourists dying on Concorde. Loneliness and technology get me every time, get my milk every time. Desire, also, stabs me not in the heart but on either side of the heart – but I had expected this. What I had not expected was that there should be some things that do not move me, that move my milk. Or that, sometimes, I only realise that I am moved when I feel the pain. I find myself lapsed into a memory I cannot catch, I find myself trying to figure out what it is in the room that is sad or lovely – was it that combination of words, or the look on his face? – what it is that has such a call on my unconscious attention, or my pituitary, or my alveolar cells.

There is a part of me, I have realised, that wants to nurse the stranger on the bus. Or perhaps it wants to nurse the bus itself, or the tree I see through the window of the bus, or the child I once was, paying my fare on the way home from school. This occasional incontinence is terrifying. It makes me want to shout – I am not sure what. Either, Take it! or, Stop! If the world would stop needing then my body would come back to me. My body would come home.

I could ask (in a disingenuous fashion) if this is what it is like to be bothered by erections. Is this what it is like to be bothered by tears? Whatever – I think we can safely say that when we are moved, it is some liquid that starts moving: blood, or milk, or salt water. I did not have a very tearful pregnancy, mostly because we don't have a television. Pregnant women cry at ads for toilet tissue: some say it is the hormones, but I think we have undertaken such a great work of imagining, we are prone to wobble on the high wire. Of course, the telly has always been a provoker of second-hand tears as well as second-hand desire. Stories, no matter how fake, produce a real biological response in us, and we are used to this. But the questions my nursing body raises are more testing to me. Do we need stories in order to produce emotion, or is an emotion already a story? What is the connection, in other words, between narrative and my alveolar cells?

I suspect, as I search the room for the hunger by the fireplace, or the hunger in her cry, that I have found a place before stories start. Or the precise place where stories start. How else can I explain the shift from language that has happened in my brain? This is why mothers do not write, because motherhood happens in the body, as much as the mind. I thought childbirth was a sort of journey that you could send dispatches home from, but of course it is not – it *is* home. Everywhere else now, is 'abroad'.

A child came out of me. I cannot understand this, or try to explain it. Except to say that my past life has become foreign to me. Except to say that I am prey, for the rest of my life, to every small thing.

Damn.

Nine Months

Day One: Ah

Development (the baby)

I WAKE UP to the sound of my baby saying, 'Ah.' It is the morning after she was born. 'Ah.' She says it clear and true. This is her voice. It sounds slightly surprised at itself. It certainly surprises me. 'Ah.' There she goes again.

Perhaps it is a reflex, the way this baby will stride across the sheet when you set her feet on the bed. She already knows how to talk, but it will be some months before she stops teasing me, and does it again.

We are born knowing everything.

Regression (me)

I wake up to the sound of my baby saying, 'Ah.' It is the morning after she was born. 'Ah.' She says it clear and true. This is her voice. It sounds slightly surprised at itself. It certainly surprises me. 'Ah.' There she goes again.

She should be crying, but she is talking instead; experimenting with this sound that comes out of her mouth. The womb is so silent. And of course. Of course! It is obvious! I have given birth to a perfect child.

I look into the cot and watch for a while. Then I decide that I must have another baby immediately.

You see, I never believed, until just this moment, that I could do this, that it could be done. Now I know that it is true – something as simple as sex can make something as complicated as a baby, a real one, and I think, What a great trick! and I wonder, How soon? How soon can we do the impossible again?

It is now the end of June. With a bit of luck we can start again in the middle of August. We could have another one by . . . next May. Allow three months for trying and failing – latest, I'll be in labour again by August of next year. Which means that I'll have to write that novel in five months, proofs at Christmas, to rush for publication late spring, and then, pop, another baby! Perfect. It all fits. I have to ring Martin and tell him this. I pick up the mobile phone he has left for me by the bedside and I dial a three. I cancel and try a six. I cancel again. I can't remember our phone number.

Usually, it takes me three years to write a book, but that's no problem: I can make babies, for heaven's sake, novels are a doddle. Look, it is all there in my head. I can flick through the pages and know the shape of it: I can relish the tone.

Usually, it takes me three years to write a book, but that's no problem: I can make babies, for heaven's sake, novels are a doddle

The novel is in my head but the phone number is not in my head. I look around the room and have a think. It's in my file – of course it is. There: just under my name. I follow the numbers with my finger and dial.

I used to be good at numbers. My brain must have been reconfigured during the night, somehow. I had heard that motherhood makes you stupid, maybe this is what they meant. Never mind, I can always use a phone book. I can do anything. I can conceive a child in the middle of November, say the 12th or 13th – Is that mid-week? It would probably be more relaxed if I ovulated at a weekend. I must ask Martin to get down the calendar.

He answers the phone.

The First Month: Dream-time

Development (*the baby*)

We dream, in our first weeks, more than at any other time in our lives. More than all the rest of our dreams over the whole span of our days. Constant dreaming. I wonder if she knows that she is awake. She opens her eyes and the world is there, she closes them and it is still there – or something very like it: the long shift of light and darkness that is week one, week two, week three. The landscape of her mother's breast. The earthquake of her mother's rising out of bed. The noise of it all.

Two faces. Two people grinning, singing, cooing, calling to her. They gaze into her eyes – but *deep* into her eyes and they do not look away. They smile – a massive break in the O of the face. Hello. Yes. Hello. Something blanks out in her head and she turns away.

Overload. Shut-down.

Regression (*me*)

I never feel her skin. She is always dressed – another vest, another babygro, always snowy white, then yellowing at the neck from crusted milk. I change her all the time, but bit by bit. I change the nappy and then the vest. Nothing will persuade me to give her a bath. She has no fat yet, under this skin of hers. So much of what we think of as skin, the pleasure of it, the way it runs under our fingers, is actually fat. Merciful, sweet fat.

I was looking forward to the softness of her, and I thought her skin would look so new. But it looks as though it belongs to someone who has been in the bath too long. It is too thin. Seven layers of cells, that is what I remember from school – our surface is seven cells thick. But I think she has only three or four. I think she has only one. It is not so much a skin, as a glaze.

At the weekend, in my parents' house, my mother quite tactfully clears the room. Just in time. I weep like someone who has been in a car crash. I weep like someone who has woken up from a dream, to find that it is all true, after all.

'Have a good cry,' says my mother, for the first time in twenty-five years. She too, at last, on home ground.

The Second Month

Development (*the baby*)

The books (the books!) say that her hands will uncurl this month, but they have always been open. Open and large and long. On the day she was born, her father looked at them and said, in a deeply regretful way, 'You know we're going to have to get a piano, now.'

She lies on her back on the white bed, wearing a white babygro, and she twists her hands slowly in front of her face; utterly graceful. She does it when there is music playing, looking very ancient, and centred, and Chinese.

She still sleeps, most of the time.

THE BABY WAKES with a yelp of hunger, and she goes for the breast like a salty old dog. 'Aaarh,' goes her mouth, as she roots to one side. 'Aaarh.' She turns away from it to fill a nappy – which is serious work, of permanently uncertain outcome, or so it seems to her; always surprising, and bravely undertaken.

'Oh, good girl!'

We squeak toys on her tummy and smile, before she blanks out, or closes her eyes to sleep again. And then one day, she does not blank out. She smiles.

Regression (*me*)

I am still not walking so well and the blood is an absolute nuisance. I look up the Internet to try and find someone who knows when this is supposed to stop, but it's all about joy and despair, it's all feeding and postnatal depression and not a single thing about leakage, seepage, anaemia. Never mind.

In the first weeks, some book tells me, I am supposed to take three baths a day. Hah! I run a bath and the water goes cold before I have a chance to get into it. I sit in a bath and then lurch like a big wet cow out of the bath, carefully, carefully over the tiles, to run to the baby. What does the baby want? We are all agreed that this is a very contented baby, but it seems, all the same, that ten minutes away from this contented baby is one minute too many. Here, darling, here's your big, wet Ma.

Actually I don't mind the bath so much, a quick dip is fine, I don't really need clean hair. I can't go out anyway, because my feet are still too big for all my shoes, except for one pair of floppy, disgusting sneakers. I don't mind that either. If I made a list of the things I cannot do, it would start and finish with going to the toilet. I never thought of going to the toilet as a fundamental human right, but I do now. It should be in some UN Charter, the opportunity and the privacy, the biological ability to go to the toilet. No one mentions this on the Internet. They talk about sex instead. Sex. Crikey.

At the recommended time, we try a bit of sex. It's a

wasteland down there. Women are awful liars. I do not think of all the women who gave birth in pain any more, I think of all the women who conceived in pain; the Irish families with eleven months between one child and the next. Did they feel the way I do, now – and then get pregnant again? No wonder they didn't tell us anything – those lowered voices in the kitchen when I was a child. Welcome to the big secret – it hurts.

But I really cannot believe that it hurts like this for everyone. Maybe I am too old. Maybe it is the fact that I have very loose joints. I think it isn't the tissue that hurts so much as the bones.

I don't know. I have never heard anyone discussing how long the pain is supposed to last. So I draw upon however many ghastly generations of suffering have preceded me and when I go back for my check-up, I smile hugely and say that everything is fine, wonderful, marvellous. I don't want to piss on the parade, and besides, it is true: I am extravagantly happy – messy, creaky, bewildered, exhausted, and in pain, but happy, hopeful, and immensely refreshed by it all.

Meanwhile, Martin is still on paternity leave and I can sleep. I have a talent for it. I doze, I nap, I snooze. I have no problem doing this. For the first time in months, I have an easy dream life – it seems my unconscious has relaxed. If the baby cries, on the other hand, I shoot up in the bed like an electrocuted corpse. Never mind the empty husk of your discarded body – pregnancy doesn't stop once they are out. I am still attached to this baby, I still feed myself in order to feed her. The only difference is the distance between us, now – all that space and air to get through. Air that she can suck in, and then exhale.

The baby cries. She cries on Saturday and also on Sunday. She does not take a break on Sunday night. And on Monday morning she cries again. We become acquainted with the long reaches of the night.

There are two, exactly opposite, ways to describe all this, and so I start to train myself in. The baby is a happy baby, I say, and lo! it is true. If I said the opposite, then this would become true instead. The baby is cranky, we will never sleep again – I would spiral downwards and the baby (the family! the house!) would be dragged down with me. So the baby is a happy baby because we have no other option, and the more we say it, the more true it becomes.

Besides. Look.

Such a beautiful, beautiful baby.

Once, maybe twice a day, I get an image of terrible violence against the baby. Like a flicker in the corner of my eye, it lasts for a quarter of a second, maybe less. Sometimes it is me who inflicts this violence, sometimes it is someone else. Martin says it is all right – it is just her astonishing vulnerability that works strange things in my head. But I know it is also because I am trapped, not just by her endless needs, but also by the endless, mindless love I have for her. It is important to stay on the right side of a love like this. For once, I am glad I am an older mother. I don't panic. I put a limit on the images that flash across my mind's eye. I am allowed two per day, maybe three. If I get more than that, then it's off to the doctor for the happy pills. Shoes or no shoes.

The Third Month

Development (*the baby*)

The baby cries for three days, on and off, and then she does something new, or she does a number of new things, all at once. She starts to grab and she also discovers her mouth, running her tongue around her lips. Or she finds her toes and starts to babble, both at the same time. The crying stops.

I wonder what was happening, for those three days? Waking up and crying, or turning and crying – seeing, reaching, scrabbling and suddenly setting up a wail. Brain fever. Hints and premonitions. Her mind is pulling itself up by its own bootstraps. There is something she must do, and she does not know what it is. Something is within reach, and she does not know what it might be. She has never done any of this before, and yet she knows that she has to do it. The shift and pressure of it must be huge. And then, all of a sudden, she breaks through. Not only 'habwabwa' but also toes! Not only this, but the other thing!

So that's what it was. What a relief.

Babies always know they have achieved something. They are naturally proud of themselves. She has a new expression every day now. Her worried look is more worried, her smile is slow, and complex, and huge.

Regression (*me*)

Somewhere in this month I realise that the baby will live, that when I wake up she will still be breathing.

From one day to the next, she changes from a tiny, mewling creature into the proper baby she is. All those old-fashioned words now apply: bonny, dandle, gurgle, dimple, posset. I give in to my stubbornly large feet, and buy new shoes.

I walk the streets of Dublin with the baby in a sling and everyone smiles at me and at my child. 'Isn't he lovely?' they say, assuming, for some reason, it is a boy. A man leans towards me on the bus. 'It's very hot,' he says. 'I have some water, ma'am, if you'd like to sponge the baby down.'

At home, Martin puts on her babygro, limb by tiny limb. 'Where did Napoleon put his armies?' he says. 'In his sleevies!'

I watch them and think how impossible it all is. I cannot see how this baby will grow into a person, any old person – a person like you, or me, or your boss, or that middle-aged woman in the street. I cannot see where it all goes.

The Fourth Month

Development (*the baby*)

The baby is becoming herself. Every day she is more present to us. A personality rises to the surface of her face, like
a slowly developing Polaroid. She frowns for the first time,
and it looks quite comical – the deliberate, frowny nature
of her frown.

Or maybe she is disappearing. There was something so
essential about her when she was just a tiny scrap: something astonishing and tenacious and altogether herself.

The baby disappears into her own personality. She gets
rounder. Her features begin to look strangely confined,
like a too-small mask in the middle of her big, round face.

It is now that babies look like Queen Victoria or Win-
ston Churchill, or anyone fat, and British, and in charge.
She is most imperious when her father picks her up. She
sits in his arms and looks over at me as if to say, So who
are you?

Regression (*me*)

The baby sits in her father's arms and looks over at me,
like I am a stranger, walked in off the street. Oh, that
blank stare. It makes me laugh, and go over to her, and
take her back from him.

Silly baba.

When I have her safe, I look at Martin, and sometimes

I recognise the wan feeling that men get, after a baby is born.

I spend the next while renegotiating this new, triangular love, with its lines of affection and exclusion. I try to make it whole. The thing I have to remember is that love is, in general, a good thing (though it often feels terrible, to me). I can see why people panic about all this: they panic about their partners being lost to them, or they panic about their babies being lost to them. Men, mostly – but not just men. Whoever is most the child in the relationship is the one who is most displaced.

I think that means me.

So, for a while I try to be, and am, that 'Mother' thing – the one who holds everyone, even myself, and keeps us safe. The container (the old bag, my dear, the old bag).

The Fifth Month

Development (the baby)

The baby looks, not at her fluffy toys' faces, eyes, ears or bits of ribbon, but at the label stitched into a seam. They all have one – a big disproportional loop of washing instructions and warnings about flammability. She likes the intricacy of the writing, but perhaps in an endlessly variable world, she is attracted to something constant and small. So much for her blue heffalump with the red feet, so much for her squeaky pink mouse – let's stick to Surface Wash Only, and the importance of 40 degrees.

Regression (*me*)

We bring the baby to America, on a book tour. Feeding her in a coffee shop, changing her nappy on the side of the road. Everywhere I travel, I think of refugees, and all the millions of women with babies in their arms, desperate for the next safe place. There is a sixteen-year-old girl in Bosnia who lives in my head, and she is doing this job just as well as I am, with as much tenderness and as much fear.

The book tour goes all right. I think.

I FLY TO Toronto and the baby goes home with her father. It doesn't occur to me to feel guilty. I drink my head off. I lactate a little mournfully into hotel sinks and make jokes about Baileys Irish Cream. I have a brilliant time (and I walk back in the door shaking like a lover).

Finished feeding, I go back on the cigarettes. I am addicted to nicotine, but I am also addicted to slipping away for two minutes every hour, and being alone. Just two minutes, maybe three. The cigarettes are in a closed room, and the ashtray is beside my computer. When she is asleep, I work. I think I am becoming addicted to working, too.

I am amazed at how much I have done. The baby sleeps for hours at a time, and I can't exactly leave the flat. So I might as well sit and type. All kinds of stuff. It doesn't look stupid to me – maybe that comes later, after you spend a few thousand hours saying, 'Look at the BLUE balloon.' So I write even faster, to outrun my fate.

The baby sleeps, and I am free. I have not so much left the human race, as just left the *race* – which suits my kind of work very well. I feel sorry for all the parents who earn their money in the real world and have to go back out there again. If you spend a few months away from the game – the shopping, shagging, striving game – then it must be hard to see the point of it, quite.

I start a short story, a woman who says, '*There is a lull, a sort of hopelessness that comes over women just before they have children, or so it was with me. I did not know where it came from. Perhaps it came from my body, perhaps it came from my life, but I had the feeling that what I was doing was no good, or that I was no good at it. I have seen other women sink suddenly like this, they lose confidence, they dither, and then, shortly afterwards, they have children.*'

Is this true?

The child sleeps. I write about a woman on a ship, with a baby in her belly. Travelling on.

The Sixth Month

Development (*the baby*)

The baby has discovered locomotion (and frustration), propelling herself on her nappied bum, on her back, across the room. I experience dread. I cannot bring the toy to her, I cannot help her to the toy. There is a lot of grunting. I wait until it reaches a certain pitch, and give in.

She is no sooner in my arms than she is scrabbling around to reach whatever thing I have not noticed was there in the first place. The world is chock-full of ignored objects, for which the baby has no filter. A discarded CD case, a packet of seeds, a tweezers, a notebook. I am worn out and amazed by her constant ambient, grazing attention, as she flings herself from me to get at one thing or another, obliging me to catch her, time and again. The world is a circus and I am her trapeze, her stilts, her net. Not just mother, also platform and prosthesis. I'm not sure I feel like a person, any more.

I think I feel a little used.

Regression (me)

In the run-up to Christmas we take the baby out, and everyone says she is the image of her father. 'I'm not a woman,' I say, 'I'm a photocopier.' But Martin is delighted to have a little version of himself, spookily female, in his arms. When I complain, he laughs and says, 'You were just the venue.'

I am a cheap drunk. Two glasses of mulled wine and I am completely squiffy, going around the room asking, 'When does the sex thing, you know . . . get back on track?' I am conducting a straw poll. I ask the men, because they are the ones who classically complain about such things. But instead of answers, I get a pained, melancholic silence. One guy just gives me a hollow look and turns away.

No one wants to talk about sex, but they all will talk about shit. Endlessly. The shit that came out both ends at once, the shit that came out the neck of the babygro, the hard round shit and the shit that is soft and green. There is nothing new parents don't know about this substance. It makes me wonder why human beings bother with disgust, and whether we will ever be disgusted again.

ON CHRISTMAS DAY, the baby likes the wrapping paper, like every baby who has been in this house, and sat on this carpet and thrown the presents over their shoulder to eat the big, loud, crinkly pictures. Such glorious repetition. Her besotted grandmother, her uncles, cousins and aunts. And I think there is a deal of grief in all this – the family renewing itself in hope, time after time.

The Seventh Month

Development (*the baby*)

The baby's eyes change colour. They are blue, edged with navy, they are green with a smoky blue ring and, one day, amber spreads through the iris. Is this you? Are these your final eyes?

I LIFT THE baby over the threshold and carry her around the new house. She loves the way one room unfolds into

another, and greets each space with delight. She leans forward, greedy for the fact that corners exist and there is
always something else around them. She sits on the floor
and likes the echo, and shouts.

Regression (me)

I cannot remember this month. We have bought a house
and we are selling our flat. Or we haven't. There is a lot of
talk about bridging finance. Martin sits up late, night after
night, doing sums on scraps of paper. I cry a fair amount.
Or stop myself from crying.

I won't spend a night in the new house. It is cold, I say.
It is too far away. There is nowhere for the baby to sleep. I
am obsessed with her sleep. She will sleep in the car on
the way out to the house, but then we must leave the
house, so she can sleep on the way home.

Every day I bump the buggy down four flights of
stairs to let people view the flat, then pull it back up
four flights with the shopping hung off the handles. I
look around the flat and I think that we are selling her
entire world.

Meanwhile, I have to earn some money, and the baby
won't sleep. When Martin walks in, I hand her over, or
even push her towards him, and go to the computer, and
will not be spoken to. He must be home in the evening. I
must be home in the evening. We are both frozen. No one
moves.

It is all too much.

The Eighth Month

Development (*the baby*)

The baby is in flying form, lying on her back and just laughing and kicking for no reason. I don't know what she is laughing at. Is this a memory? Is she imagining, for the first time, tickles, even though there are no tickles there?

She may be the only truly happy person on the planet. I look at her and hope she isn't bonkers.

Regression (*me*)

I close the door on the flat, busy with removals men. I don't say goodbye.

On the way to the new house, the clutch cable snaps in the fast lane of the dual carriageway as I gear down to stop at some traffic lights. I break the lights and crawl across the road to find the kerb in a slow swerve. I ring Martin, whose mobile is on answering machine. I ring my mother and father. I run down to a local pub with the baby in my arms and ask does anyone know a local garage. That fella over there owns one, they say. I get to the garage in first gear. And so on, and so forth.

Behind me, the removals men have left the washing-machine connection leaking into the flat, a fact we do not hear about until two days later, when the water spills into the hall. We still have no car. Martin stays late after work in order to dry out the flat while I unpack cardboard boxes – or try to, while looking after the baby – and complain, complain, complain. I have no time to work, I say. I don't even have time to unpack. How does it always, always, fucking end up like this, with the woman climbing a domestic Everest while the man walks out the door? I would go out and look for a nursery, but I have to start earning before I can pay for a nursery. I have to start earning to pay for the house.

There is a freak snowstorm. We have no milk. I put the baby in the buggy and, slithering along the path, I push her through the gale.

The Ninth Month

Development (*the baby*)
Spring. The child looks out into the garden at the changing light. There is something about this scene that she understands and I don't know what it is. I don't know if it is the tree – the fact that the tree is there, or that it is green, or that it is made of so many leaves. I do not know if it is the wind she likes, the way the tree moves when it blows. She raises her hand and starts to shout. It is a long, complicated shout, 'Aah aaah bleeh oh. Ahh nyha mang bwah!' She is making a speech. Her hand is lifted high; the palm reaches towards the sky as she declaims. As far as I can tell there is nothing she wants in the garden, she just

wants to say that it is there, and that it is good. She wants to say this loudly and at length.

The baba bears witness. The baba testifies.

Regression (*me*)

I have no notes for this month.

I unpack boxes. I hold the baby and love her, like a tragic event. She loves me like the best joke out.

On the day she is nine months old, I think that she has been outside of me, now, for just as long as she was inside. She is twice as old.

I am the mirror and the hinge. There she is. She is just as old as herself.

Time

MY EARLIEST MEMORY is of a pot stand. It is set into a corner with a cupboard on one side and, on the other, a shallow step. This is where my head begins. The step leads to another room, and far on the other side of the room, there is a white-haired woman sitting in a chair.

Discussions with my mother lead to just one pot stand, in a seaside cottage the summer I was eighteen months old. It was, she says, made of black iron and it stood beside a real step and the white-haired woman must be her own mother who died when I was six. This image of her is all that I have, and even then it is not so much an image as a sense. She may have been asleep, but I think she was reading. And there was something very quiet and covert about the pot stand, which was a pyramid affair with shelves for four pots. I can remember a little saucepan on the top shelf. I am tempted to say that there was a big saucepan on the bottom one, but this is pushing things a bit. I would give anything to remember what the lino was like.

At nine months, the baby puts her head in a pot and says, Aaah Aaah Aaah. She says it very gently and listens to the echo. She has discovered this all by herself. By way of celebration, I put my own head into the pot and say, Aaah Aaah Aaah. Then she does it again. Then I do it again. And so on.

The rest of my family don't believe that I remember the pot stand, on the grounds that it is a stupid memory and, anyway, I was far too young. It is the job of families to reject each other's memories, even the pleasant ones, and being the youngest I am sometimes forced to fight for the contents of my own head. But my brother broke his elbow that summer. My mother had to take him to hospital in Dublin and my grandmother looked after us while she was away. This was the first time in my life that I was without my mother for any length of time. If she had stayed, then I am certain that I would not have remembered anything at all of that house – not the pot stand, and not my grandmother either.

We pilfer our own memories, we steal them from the world and salt them away.

I first left the baby when she was four months old. Some of the days when I was away, she spent with my mother. I wonder what image might remain with her from that time: a colour, a smell, a combination of shapes perhaps, affectless and still – and in the distance, someone. Just that. Someone.

And in the foreground? The carpet perhaps. I hope she

remembers my parents' carpet, the one I remember as a child, with a pattern of green leaves like stepping-stones all the way down the hall.

I have another, possibly earlier, memory of pulling the wallpaper off the wall from between the bars of my cot. My mother is absent from this scene too, but though the Pot Stand Memory is neither happy nor unhappy, this one is quite thrilling. I almost certainly ate the paper. The plaster underneath it was pink and powdery, and I imagine now that I can remember the shivery taste of it. I also remember the shape of the tear on the wall, or I think I do. At any rate, I see it in my mind's eye – a seam on the left, stunningly straight, with four gammy strips pulled away, like a fat raggedy set of fingers, on the right.

I know this memory is, in some sense, true, but when I try to chase it, it disappears. It exists in peripheral vision, and presents itself only when I focus on something else – like typing, for example. When I stop writing this sentence and look up from the screen to try to see the pattern of the wallpaper – a blank. Memories, by their nature, may not be examined, and the mind's eye is not the eye we use, for example, to cross the road.

I wonder if this is the way that the baby sees things: vaguely and all at once. I imagine it to be a very emotional way to exist in the world. Perhaps I am being romantic – but the visual world yields nothing but delight to her. There are (it seems) no horrors, no frights. Tiny babies see only in monochrome. I imagine colour leaking into her head like a slowly adjusted screen – tremendously slow, like a vegetable television growing silently in the corner of the room. I imagine her focus becoming sharper and deeper, like some infinitely stoned cameraman adjusting his lens. 'Oh,' she says – or something that is the precursor to 'Oh', a shallow inhalation, a stillness as she is caught by something, and begins to stalk it: careful, rapt – the most beautiful sound in the world: the sound of a baby's wondering breath.

Something pulls in me when she is caught like this. For months I am a slave to her attention. The world is all colour, light and texture and I am her proud companion. I have no choice. None of us do. In a café, three women look over to smile at her, and then, as one, they look up. 'Oh, she likes the light,' says one, and this fact pleases us all. Immensely.

The light, of course, is horrible, and this is one of the reasons mothers think they are losing their minds: this pride in the baby looking at the light, this pride in the light as they introduce it to the baby, 'Yes, the light!' There is a certain zen to it; the world simple and new as we all stop to admire the baby admiring a wrought-iron candelabra with peculiar dangly bits and five – yes, five! – glowing, tulip-shaped bulbs.

She is years away from knowing what 'five' might be, but maybe she already gets the 'fiveness' of it. This is the way her eyes move: One, one more! Another one! All of them! The other two. The first one again, another one! Something else.

Sometimes she holds her hand up like the baby Christ, and looks as though she contains everything, and understands it all. I do not ask to be forgiven, but still I feel redemption in the completeness of her gaze. And I feel the redemption in her fat baby wrists and her infinitely fine, fat baby's hand. The baby is a blessing, but sometimes she does, she *must*, also bless, which is to say that she simply sees, and lifts her hand, as a sign.

I pick the baby up and we look in the wardrobe mirror, which has always been for her a complicated delight: What is it? It's a baby! She smiles, it smiles back! (Complication upon complication! It's me! It's me! she says, and all her synapses, as I imagine, going ping! ping! ping!) She sees me smiling at her in the mirror; she sees her mother turning to smile at her in the room, and oh, it's too much, she lunges forwards to examine the knob on the wardrobe door.

There are actually two knobs on the wardrobe. One is wooden and the other, for some reason, is an amber-coloured plastic. The baby goes from one to the other and back again. One of the first confusions in her young life was when myself and Martin both looked at her at the same time: 'Oh no, there's two of them.' It almost felt unfair.

As she grew older, there was nothing she liked more than to be held by one of us and to look at the other, in a somewhat haughty way. Older still, she is completely content when the two of us are with her, quietly in a room. She has travelled from one, to two, perhaps to many. I think of this as she goes from the wooden knob to the amber one – a fairy tale of sameness and difference. This one. That one.

Of course, the first difference between this and the other is not between mother and father, or even between baby and 'baby in the mirror', but between one breast and . . . the other! If women had five teats, then mankind might, by now, be living on the moon.

Yesterday, it was warm, and I took off her socks and stood her on the grass. She loved this, but maybe not so much as I did – her first experience of grass. For her, this green stuff was just as different and as delicious as everything else – the 'first' was all mine. Sometimes, I feel as though I am introducing her to my own nostalgia for the world.

In the meantime, grass is green and springy and amazingly multiple and just itself. It might even be edible. Everything goes into her mouth. This is the taste of yellow. This is the taste of blue. Since she started moving about she has also experienced the taste of turf, of yesterday's toast, and probably of mouse droppings, because it was weeks before I realised we were not alone in the house. Paper remains her ultimate goal, and she looks over her shoulder now to check if I am around. That wallpaper looks nice.

My own mother, who is curator and container of many things, among them the memory of my pot stand, worries that she is getting forgetful. The distant past is closer all the time, she says. If this is true, then the memory of her own mother is getting stronger now; sitting in a house by the sea, surrounded by children who are variously delighted, or worried, or concentrating on other things.

When you think about it, the pots can't have stayed there for long. I would have pulled them down. There would have been noise, though my memory of them is notably, and utterly, silent. Perhaps what I remember is the calm before a chaos of sound and recrimination. That delicious, slow moment, when a baby goes very, very quiet, knowing it is about to be found out.

The other morning, the baby (silently) reached the seedlings I have under the window, and she filled her mouth with a handful of hardy annuals and potting compost. I tried to prise her mouth open to get the stuff out. She clamped it shut. She bit me (by accident). She started to cry. When she cried, her mouth opened. She was undone by her own distress and this seemed so unfair to me that I left her to it. I hadn't the heart. Besides, it said on the pack that the compost was sterilised.

But she will not let my finger into her mouth, now, even to check for a tooth (she is very proud of her teeth), and when she clamps it shut and turns away she is saying, 'Me,' loud and clear. 'Oh,' a friend said, when she started to crawl, 'it's the beginning of the end,' and I knew what she meant. It is the beginning of the end of a romance between a woman who has forgotten who she is and a child who does not yet know.

Until one day there will come a moment, delightful or banal, ordinary or strange, that she will remember for the rest of her life.

Advice

IT IS THE middle of the morning – an ordinary morning of undressing, dressing, sterilising, mixing, spooning, wiping, squawking, smiling, banging, reaching for the bread knife, falling down, climbing up, in the middle of which – a crisis! which is dealt with in the military style: change nappy, remove shitty vest, wash hands, find clean vest, pull baby away from stairs, comfort baby when she cries for stairs, dress baby, lift shitty vest, soak shitty vest, wash hands, and finally we are out the door and into the car seat, off to the supermarket, me singing 'Twinkle Twinkle Little Star' and remembering I have left the back door wide open. I am driving carefully. The sun is shining. I think, What will I tell her when she grows up? Actually I think, What if I die? What if I die, now, soon, or even later on? I am in the throes of car accidents and chemotherapy, between the first twinkle twinkle and the second twinkle twinkle. By the fourth repetition, she is trying to dress herself for school and wandering out of the house alone.

Her father has disappeared from this fantasy. She is facing the wide world, and there is nothing I can do to help her. I cannot reach her, I cannot speak. I should write her a letter, but what could it say?

Park, take the baby out of car seat, try to find keys, put the baby back in car seat, find keys, take the baby out of car seat, lock car, and so on, all the way through the coin for the trolley (leave baby down on the ground? Is that dog shit? Who would have thought there could be so much shit in the world?), I am banishing foolish thoughts. They are just the big metaphysics, swooping over our small, lovely life. I must try to live in the middle, think in a mid-dling way, and so, as we sail along the aisles, as I keep hold of her arm while ducking down, over and over again, to pick up the half-chewed, as yet unpaid-for banana that she enjoys throwing out of the trolley, I concentrate on a sim-pler task. Advice. What advice can you give a child to arm and protect them in the world? I am not thinking of *Don't talk to strangers*, but of the things that only I would say. This is the perk that every mother demands, somewhere along the line – to exercise her own, particular personal-ity. Usually, let's admit it, with disastrous results.

Smile at the checkout, apologise for the banana, sing, 'Do You Love an Apple,' to keep her still in the paused trolley, search busily through my empty head, only one nugget comes to mind. *Beware of modest people. They are the worst megalomaniacs of all.*

For the rest of the day (scrub out the shitty vest? No,

throw out the shitty vest. Don't tell anyone), this is the only wisdom I can find, the only sentence, *Beware of modest people . . .* of course it is true: Einstein, Mother Teresa, some women I know, many many nuns, a couple of poets – all so lovely, all so monstrous. You have to have a very big ego to wrestle it down to something so small. I know, I've tried. *Beware the tender smile, my daughter, the love that saddens, the crinkly eyes . . .*

But it isn't exactly useful, as advice goes. Not as useful as *Don't touch the oven, it is hot!* which is what I spend my day saying, now. *Hot! Hot!* I would also say, *Dirty! Dirty!* but I can't be bothered. I concentrate on *Careful!* or *Gently!* or plain *NO!* And so it will be, for years yet. The first thousand days of her life, the whole remarkable world around her, and all that I have to say could be reduced to one phrase, *Proceed . . . with caution.* And for the thousand days after that? *Don't talk to strangers,* of course, which is the same thing again, in a way.

There must be more. I just can't think of anything. I open my mouth and . . . my own mother comes falling out of it. But of course.

She takes advice very seriously, my mother. She still doles it out on a regular basis. She is not afraid to repeat herself. She is often right – when, for example, she says to me, *You should flatter people a little. You should at least try.*

I never listened to a word of it; except maybe for, *If Joyce was worried about what his Mammy might say, he would never have written* Ulysses (a piece of advice which she has paid for, many times since), or the excellent, *Never use a big word where a small word will do*. What about, *Cheer up, we'll soon be dead*? Did she really say that? Of course she would deny it, now – though I still find it giddily bleak and quite useful. *Cheer up, we'll soon be dead*, just one of her variations on the mother's mantra of, *All this will pass*. Having the wrong pencil-case, being forced to share a desk with Brenda Dunne, losing the boy you love, *In fifty years' time you might even laugh about it* (but what happens, Ma, when you run out of time?)

Never laugh at someone's religion, that's a good one. Actually, what she said was, 'If someone worships a stone in the road and you laugh at them, they will pick it up and hit you with it.' Fair enough.

I didn't start arguing with her until it came to men. *Never humiliate a man in public* – intriguing, this one. What were you to do in private? And then again, some men are very easily humiliated. They are humiliated when you are clever, and it is hard work being stupid. They are humiliated if you flirt, or if you don't flirt. You could spend your life tending to some man's pride, but, *There is no excuse for marrying a bastard*, she said, or something like it, as if falling for the wrong man was just a lazy way to go about your life, when there were so many good men in the world. In those days, a Good Man was someone who allowed the household the use of his pay-packet, who wasn't a drunk, and who didn't hit you. Actually, this is probably still a good baseline. Maybe this is something I could pass on to my daughter. I could translate it as:

Never sleep with someone who has more problems than you – 50 per cent of people fail to follow this advice, and it is vital to be in the other half. What else?

Never trust someone beyond their strength, because – oh, my darling girl, and the million things that could hurt her; not strangers, but friends, because these are the ones who break your heart – she must arm herself against the weak more than the strong . . .

'Oh, get a grip, Mother.'

All advice is useless. *Don't wear patterns next to your face. Never plant camellias facing east. Have sex before you go out for the night, not after you come home. The things that make you fat are booze and biscuits – nothing else.* What about, *Earn money* – my mother used to tell me to do this all the time. All right. *Earn money* – you must overcome the natural distaste you might feel for cash. If you dislike the system, then find a crack in it, and live there. And the simplest way to earn money is to go out and earn it. That is what is called the (middle-class) Tao of money.

I didn't listen to that either.

And look at this baby, just look at her – with her steady baby's gaze; her serious baby's eyes that have some joke in them all the same, as she putters towards the plastic shopping bags.

'No!' I shout, and when she cries I say, 'It's all right. It's all right.'

Proceed with caution.

Actually, most of the time I don't know what 'No' is for. Mind the door, mind the books don't fall, mind your fingers, hot!, careful of the cup, don't touch the dirt. After one particularly long day, I decided against it. It was making me depressed. So I left her to her own devices for a while, and we all cheered up.

The Sioux, Martin tells me, let their babies learn everything for themselves: fall into the river, fall into the fire, anything. But children are quite careful, really.

And what does she say to me?

'Burr!' says the baby, pointing at the sky.

Look at the bird, Mama. This is my baby's advice to me. *Look at the bird!*

Being Two

'I'M TWO,' SHE says, standing on the bathroom scales. And indeed there it is on the dial, the nice, round-topped, swoop and swan of '2'. She is fond of being two. She is nearly three. Her new little brother is only zero with a few silly bits added on. He is not even a proper number yet.

'So how's it all going?'

I want to tell people about her, but I want to tell them *everything* about her, because there is nothing else. The proper maternal mode is gabble. The proper maternal instrument is the phone. We are all a Jewish joke.

'She can read! She read her name on her birthday card!'

'And what about the number?'

'No problem. Twenty-one.'

And I want to tell them nothing about her. She is a child, she must not be described. She must be kept fluid and open; not labelled or marked. I could say that she is playful, open, stubborn, bossy, winsome, serious, giddy, boisterous, clinging, gorgeous – but these are words that describe every single two-year-old on the planet, they are not the essence of herself, the thing that will always be there. Describing a child is a matter of prediction or nostalgia. There is no present moment. You are always trying to grasp something that changes even as you look at it. Besides, all children are the same, somehow. And still I know she is different from the general run of toddlers. How do I know? I just do. And if you think I am biased, this is what other people have said about her:

'There's no doubt about it, she is a fabulous child.'
Donal Enright, Grandfather.

'I have to say I never met a more interesting, or nicer, two-year-old.'
Theo Dombrowski, a friend.

'She is very advanced for two, and I should know – I am an educational psychologist.'
*Stranger (possibly mad), in the foyer
of a West Cork hotel.*

'Oh, all her geese are swans,' my mother used to say about boastful mothers.

In the old days – as we call the 1970s, in Ireland – a mother would dispraise her child automatically. I understand this urge: you don't want a toddler to get the edge on you, especially when you are trying to get them past a shop full of sweets; so 'She's a monkey,' a mother might say, or 'Street angel, home devil,' or even my favourite, 'She'll have me in an early grave.'

It was all part of growing up in a country where praise of any sort was taboo. Of course we are nicer now, we are more confident and positive and relaxed – which does not explain the strange urge I had when a man looked at her photograph. 'Such lovely eyes,' he said, and I said, 'Oh, they're all right,' or something even worse. It is true that I felt acutely, burningly praised, but I also felt the deep hiss of a mother who reaches out her hand to say, *Give me back my baby*.

People don't write much about their children. Sometimes they say it is to protect the child's privacy – but I am not sure how private a ten-year-old feels, for example, about a picture of his two-year-old self, or how connected. I think it is simpler than that. I think people don't want to write about their children because they think that, if they do, their children might die. And that's just for starters. I think they do not want to surrender any part of their children, certainly not for money, and particularly not to a crowd.

So this is just a mock-up. It is not the real girl at all.

'YOU HAVE A smelly bum.'

'Go away. Go smell your own bum.'

'I can't smell my bum. I can't get my face around.'

She already loves a paradox, and most of them are

anatomical. 'A shark has a long nose so he can't see his mouth,' she says (well, you know what she means). Which reminds me, I must get her *Alice in Wonderland*, though:

'That's me,' she said, a while ago.

'Where?'

'In that car.'

'Oh. You're in that car?'

'Yes.'

'Where are you going?'

'I going to my house.'

'Where is your house? What kind of house?'

'It has a yellow door.'

'Oh.'

After a while, I say, 'And what is your name?'

'Alice,' she says.

This spooked me no end. She is not called Alice, and we do not have a yellow (or lello) door. I thought she was having a past-life regression, there in the back of the car – well, I didn't really, but sometimes I wish I was that bit more credulous. Then later, in the bath, she was all talk of rabbits and my-ears-and-whiskers, and I realised that she had heard, or seen, her first ever *Alice in Wonderland*.

Fantastic. The rabbit went down the plug hole, in the end.

Her father must have been away if I was giving her a bath – these more intriguing dialogues happen when her ordinary life is unbalanced in some way.

'I love him,' she says, pointing at the picture of the

author on the back of one of her books. Colin McNaughton, he is called – a very pleasant, handsome-looking guy. I have to admire her taste, though the writer thing is a bit unsettling. Never fall for a writer, I want to say. Never, ever, ever make that mistake.

Instead I say, 'Oh.'

'Yes. Because my Dada is away.'

This is nothing (I flatter myself) to the anxiety she feels when her mother is away. Endlessly recounted is the story of the witch in the supermarket, last Hallowe'en. A woman in a mask who came up and, I presume, cackled at her while she was sitting in the trolley and then, when the child started to cry, took off the witch's mask to show that she was only a nice person underneath. Silly bitch. I think taking the mask off made it worse, but there you go; I suppose it's too late to sue. Later that evening, she stood with her father in the dark, watching the local fireworks from an upstairs window. When I came home, there were spent rockets in the flower-beds.

A hundred renditions of the witch-in-the-supermarket story later, I hit on the key. I was away at the time – does she remember? She certainly does. She remembers that I was in Paris. What was I doing in there? she suddenly asks, Was I frightened? Was I watching the fireworks, too?

'I was,' I say, and once I am placed in the picture – somewhere on the other side of the fireworks – the story is allowed to fade. But she is still obsessed by witches, which is presumably, somehow, my fault – also bad fairies and wicked stepmothers. There are no nice women in the old stories. Though one morning she announces a dream – a good dream. What was it about?

'Barbie,' she says, looking very coy.

'Oh? And what was Barbie doing?'

'She was reading me a book.'

Which is one of the things that I do, of course – my tendency to interpret the child mocked by an image of myself as a six-foot plastic toy. And maybe it is not all a drama of good mother / bad mother, maybe she was just angling for a Barbie and knows how much I'd love to know what happens in her dreams. She is two. She has – perhaps they all have – a delicious mind.

She has a quality, sometimes, when she is tired. Her eyes become distant, and slightly blissed. She looks at you strangely, as though she has been here before.

I am heavily pregnant and under the shower. We are alone in the house, and I think, What would happen if I fell? Would she be able to fetch the phone? I can see it all: the gravid woman, wedged into the bath, the water playing on her senseless belly, the toddler bereft, the time passing; all this flashing through my mind in a moment, while she tilts her face up to me, and says, 'Don't fall.'

Or I am going up the stairs with her in my arms. I think, I must ring my mother and she says, 'Does Granny have stairs?'

They are so tiny and inconsequential, these coincidences of mind. They always surprise me, even though they are not so surprising – after all, for most of the time we live the same life – and I begin to build a little wall against my Midwich Cuckoo. Some of my thoughts are so unbecoming. I catch myself and think, 'I hope she didn't get that one.'

All of this is very slight, you understand, and nothing you could absolutely put a finger on. It never involves a future event, but when she talks about someone, I might ring them, just to check that they are still alive. They always are.

I tell her about her Granny and Granda, how they met at a dance, in a hotel by the sea. She says, 'Was I watching?'

I am tempted to say, 'I don't know.'

What else?

She is very bossy about the world. She is always putting it in its place and sometimes there is very little difference between ordering it, and ordering it around. 'Cars don't go into houses, they are too big.' 'That car [a convertible] has no lid.' 'Cars have roofs and motor bikes have helmets.'

Yes,' I say to all this. I have to say, Yes, or she will repeat it ad infinitum. 'Yes. Yes, absolutely. Yes.'

For months we were trapped in a kind of Beckettian rhapsody, as she tried to make the world safe. From the back seat:

'Mama, cars don't go into houses, do they?'

'No, they don't.'

'Do they?'

'No, they certainly don't, they're too big.'

'And they don't go on the path.'

'No.'

'They go on the road.'

'Yes.'

'People go on the path.'

'Yes. Absolutely.'

'Where's it gone?'

'Where's what gone?'

'Where's the street light gone?'

'It's behind us.'

'But where's it gone?'

'We'll see another one.'

'But where's it gone?'

'Oh, take it easy.'

It happens on the same stretch of road – she always grieves the disappearing street lights: the way they keep coming, only to flick away.

It was around here that I once said, 'I used to work over there, before you were born.'

'When I was a baby.'

'No, before that. Before you were born.'

'When I was just a teeny-tiny baby?'

'No, before you were even here. Before you were in my tummy.'

'I was . . . Where.'

'You were just a twinkle in your Daddy's eye.'

'I not a twinkle. I NOT a twinkle!!!' And she started to

kick and squawk. I suppose I did sound a little smug; a little complacent about the idea that she was once non-existent. Too tough, really, for any age, but especially tough for two.

Her favourite story is *Sleeping Beauty*. But only recently. Fairy tales happened in the last few weeks, at the end of 'two' and the beginning of 'nearly three', because 'two' is a very long place. She started the year obsessed by gender, moved into a long toilet phase, and ended with witches, princesses, and sleep. But also in there were numbers, which gave her huge pleasure, as did all kinds of repetition and ritual and make-believe. There was also the endless amusement to be got from ordering her parents around and giving them grief.

'Not the blue cup with the straw.'

'I thought you wanted a straw.'

'I don't want a straw.'

'Do you want the blue cup?'

'I don't want a straw.'

'OK.'

'I don't want a straw!'

And so on, all the way to wails, screams, tears. Of course the dialogue is edited to make me look like a saint, which I am not. ('The cup goes in the bin. All right? The cup – see this cup? – it's going in the bin.') Months of attrition later I realise that the best thing to do is to become benignly invisible. If I can manage simply not to exist, there is no escalation.

She started the year obsessed by gender, moved into a long toilet phase, and ended with witches, princesses, and sleep

She is only two.

Though sometimes, I am two, too.

And when she has done every single, possible thing to provoke, thwart, whine, refuse, baulk, delay, complicate and annoy, I wonder how the human race survived.

'I'll swing for you,' I heard myself saying once. Which is Irish for 'I will kill you and take the consequences.'

She is two. She is *only* two.

There is nothing better than watching her play shopping. When she walks across the room to the 'shops' she does not so much walk as 'walk' with an exaggeration of hip and heel that says, 'Here I am "walking" to the shops.' She hums to the rhythm of it. Hum. Hum. Hum. Hum. Walk. Walk. Walk. Walk.

All her inverted commas are huge, and even in ordinary conversation she will sometimes use an 'other' voice; fake wise, or fake grown-up, with much use of the word 'actually'. As in, 'That looks like a duck, actually.'

There is a place on the wall where she gets things, like broccoli, or sweets, or water. She runs over to the wall and goes, 'Ssszzsst,' rolling and twiddling her hands in a 'complicated' way. Then she runs back from the wall with my imaginary cup of tea.

'Oh, *thank* you.'

Her anxiety about the baby that is on the way brings back all kinds of eating games. 'Gobble gobble nyum nyum,' she says, 'I am eating your arm.' She does not like it so much when I eat her back. 'Nyum nyum, scarf scarf gobble nyum.' She runs to her special place on the wall and takes down bits of herself, which she sticks along her arm, and pats back into place. She is getting her real arm back, she says. I have just eaten her pretend one.

'Yes,' I say, thinking, as I often do, that she is an outrageously wonderful child. Sometimes, of course, she is just outrageous.

She is two.

'Can I be two?' I say, and have a pretend tantrum on the floor. Just a small one. I lie on my back and drum my heels. She doesn't like the look of this at all.

It is a very long year. When November comes I miss the child October gave us, that paradise, when I was only moderately pregnant and potty training had not yet begun. And I miss the baby, just walking, who looked at the black and yellow stripes of the Kilkenny hurling team and said, 'Bees! Bees!'

This is the girl who was entranced by every flying thing, who followed a plane across the sky in her Granny's back garden and never took her eyes away once, whose first or second word may have been 'bird', whose first big word was 'helicopter', who can already tell a hoverfly from a bee (but not a bee from a wasp), and a tweet-tweet birdie from one that goes caw-caw. This is the girl who got 'a moth' from Santa Claus for Christmas. She is also, of course, fond of woodlice, but give her a glider, a kite, a cloud, a woman under a parachute, a fairy, or a balloon, and she will choose them over a slug or snail any day. She is close to the ground, which might be the reason that she is always looking up, but the reason she loves butterflies is the reason she likes the mirror and also the reason that she likes hands: it is that one side is the same as the other side, and nothing has given her greater joy, I think, than folding a piece of paper over some splashes of paint, and opening a Rorschach of complete delight. It is always a butterfly, because this is the best thing it could be, and other things that mirror and match are butterflies too.

'A bum is like a butterfly,' she said once.

'Yes. Yes.'

The first play she ever went to was about bees and, when the actors gave her a set of paper wings, she declared into the stillness of the audience, 'I can fly.'

Of Christ on the Cross she says, 'Are they wings?' and I say, 'No, darling, those are His arms.'

'WHEN I WAS a little baby,' she says, wrestling with the idea of growing up, now that there is another baby in Mammy's tummy.

'When I was a little baby,' she says (because these things are always said twice), 'I used to say "pine-a-cacket".'

'And what do you say now?'

'I say, "pineapple".'

We are both amused by this. We are both fond of her former self. Now she is a big girl, she looks with tenderness at a picture of herself newborn. 'Look how pleased your Dada is to see you,' I say. She looks at this for a while, and then walks over to embrace him, properly and formally. Sometimes she has astonishing emotional clarity; and I have to catch my breath at the rightness of her.

She is nearly three. She is learning, she told me, not to cry at things. I said she could still cry at some things but she shook her head. No, she would not cry. And when she is three, she says, she will not be scared of the witch in the supermarket. It is a serious business, growing up; a heavy responsibility.

On the Friday before her birthday, I bring a (pink!) cake into the crèche, and she asks, 'I'm going to have a cake, even though I am still two?' and I realise that it is not the cake, or the candles, or the party, or the presents that matter to her, so much as *being three*. It is a different place.

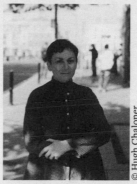
© Hugh Chaloner

ANNE ENRIGHT is one of Ireland's most celebrated writers and the current Laureate for Irish Fiction. She was born and raised in Dublin, the city where she now lives. She writes articles, essays and short stories but is most famous for her novels, in particular *The Gathering*, which won the Man Booker Prize in 2007, and her most recent, the critically acclaimed, *The Green Road*.

Anne Enright's novels are interested in the difference between romance and biology, between the love we choose, and the love to which we are helpless. She writes of family life in all its maddening, ordinary glory. *Making Babies*, from which this short book is drawn, is her only work of memoir, written before Anne Enright became an internationally renowned novelist. It was lauded for its humour and honesty. Ian Sansom wrote of it: '*Making Babies* is not just a good book, it's a good thing. It induces hope. It creates an appetite for life. It is also a very effective contraceptive'.

RECOMMENDED BOOKS BY ANNE ENRIGHT:

The Green Road
The Gathering
Making Babies

Still in love with Babies?

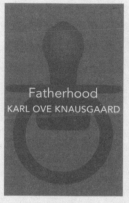

Fatherhood
KARL OVE KNAUSGAARD

VINTAGE MINIS

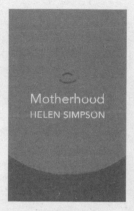

Motherhood
HELEN SIMPSON

VINTAGE MINIS

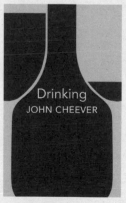

Drinking
JOHN CHEEVER

VINTAGE MINIS

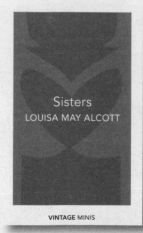

Sisters
LOUISA MAY ALCOTT

VINTAGE MINIS

VINTAGE MINIS

The Vintage Minis bring you the world's greatest writers on the experiences that make us human. These stylish, entertaining little books explore the whole spectrum of life – from birth to death, and everything in between. Which means there's something here for everyone, whatever your story.

vintageminis.co.uk